Lysergic Acid Diethylamide

LSD: Improving Lives, Psychotherapy, and the Brain.

by Gareth Hamlyn

©2016

Contents

Chapter 1: LSD

Lysergic acid diethylamide or lysergide is a hallucinogen that is taken by recreational drug users to distort reality (Quigley and Waun, 2011). LSD was discovered by Albert Hofmann, a Swiss chemist working for a pharmaceutical company, in 1938 by accident. After its discovery, the drug was used in experiments for thirty years to treat drug addictions, autism, terminal cancer, and schizophrenia. In 1965, the drug became illegal to produce, possess, and sell as a result of the Drug Abuse Control Amendment. LSD is one of the most potent psychedelic drugs, which can produce mood and perception-altering effects that last up to twelve hours with as little as thirty micrograms. The production and use of the drug in nearly every Western nation is illegal, and there has been no medically accepted use for it to date. The drug is produced through a synthetic process using ergot, which is a fungus that grows on rye grass and some grains. After synthesized, the drug is odorless, colorless, and slightly bitter-tasting, and it can be taken orally or absorbed through the skin. The drug is typically produced and distributed on drug-soaked blotter paper that can be chewed or swallowed. The drug was commonly used by teens in Western nations throughout the 1990s, and it is still presently popular today for use by individuals who attend clubs, raves, and concerts.

LSD is considered to be an extremely potent hallucinogenic drug that is typically derived from the ergot alkaloids, like ergotamine and ergonovine, and is generally prepared through chemical synthesization in laboratories (LSD, 2016). The chemical structure of LSD resembles that of other hallucinogenic drugs like bufotenine, psilocybin, harmine, and ibogaine, which all produce effects by blocking the action of serotonin transmission within the brain. The inhibition of serotonin action results in drastic deviations from normal behavior, and it was used early after its discovery as a psychotomimetic agent to induce mental states that were similar to psychotic diseases, specifically schizophrenia.

(Royal Society of Chemistry, 2015)

An image that depicts the chemical structure of LSD.

The drug alters users' perceptions by disrupting serotonin and neurotransmission in their brains, but the pharmacology and neural pathways of the drug are still not fully understood by neurologists (Quigley and Waun, 2011). Neurologists have discovered from magnetic resonance imaging that once ingested the drug primarily affects the cerebral cortex and the locus coeruleus. The cerebral cortex is an area of the brain that is involved with individuals' moods and perceptions, and the locus coeruleus is an area of the brain in which sensory signals meet from all parts of the body. LSD mimics the effects of natural hallucinogens, like mescaline and psilocybin, which have been used in both social and religious rituals in cultures throughout the world for thousands of years.

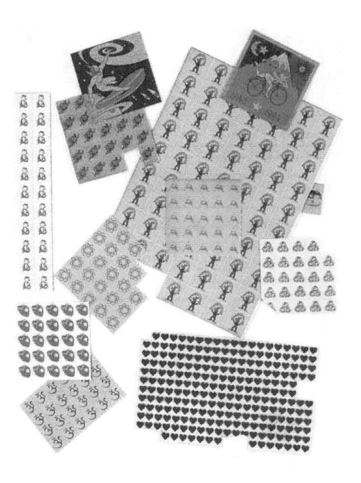

(Devianart, 2016)

LSD is typically soaked into blotter paper and sold on the black market. This allows dealers to profit from its sales, and it also assists in lessening the dose strength compared to the LSD being sold and used in the 1960s, which has resulted in less negative outcomes for users during sessions.

The effects of LSD are felt by a user within an hour after Ingestion, and they can last for up to twelve hours depending on the dosage taken (Quigley and Waun, 2011). The drug is absorbed in the intestinal tract, it circulates throughout the body and brain, it is metabolized in users' livers, and it is excreted through the urinary tract within twenty-four hours following ingestion. The psychological effects of LSD are emotional and sensory, and emotions typically shift from euphoria to confusion and despair, which is dependent on specific users and the session in which the drug is taken. LSD users have reported feeling simultaneous emotions at once in combination with increased intensity of colors, smells, and sounds. Users also report being able to see sounds and smell colors, and there is a typical loss of perception of time. Finally, some users report having out-of-body experiences and sensations, and hallucinations have caused some users to feel that their bodies have changed shape or merged with other objects in the environment in which the session has taken place. The physical effects of the drug may result in appetite loss, pupil dilation, dry mouth, palpitations, nausea, perspiration, and dizziness.

LSD can be an extremely dangerous drug when taken by individuals unknowingly or in particular environments, but it is not addictive like stimulants, opioids, alcohol, or nicotine (Quigley and Waun, 2011). The effects of the drug differ as a result of users different personalities, moods, expectations, and environments, and the drug's effects are considered to be highly unpredictable and variable in accordance with the aforementioned factors and the amount taken.

Users also report varying effects from one session to the next, and the majority of LSD-related deaths stem from panic reactions that are caused by illusions following ingestion of the drug. There are two long-term side effects that have been documented by the medical community in relation to the drug: psychosis and hallucinogen persisting perception disorder. Researchers do not fully understand why these two side effects persist in some users but not others. Psychosis has occurred in individuals who have never had psychological disorders prior to using the drug and have no family history of psychological problems. Psychosis resulting from LSD use can include mood swings, loss of both cognitive and communication skills, and hallucinations, which can last from years to decades. Also, hallucinogen persisting perception disorder or flashbacks have been reported to last for a couple of seconds to hours in some users from years to decades as well, and they involve altered vision that causes bright flashes and trails following moving objects.

The negative side effects seen from the drug are considered to be less common today because LSD that is sold on the black market y is considered to be less weaker than average dosages of the drug sold in the past (Quigley and Waun, 2011). The dose strength of LSD sold on the black market today is typically between 20 to 80 micrograms in comparison to the dose strength of the drug in the

1960s, which was between 100 to 200 micrograms. Flashbacks from former LSD use have been reported following the use of other recreational drugs such as marijuana, and there are reports that serotonin reuptake inhibitors can compound hallucinogen persisting perception disorders.

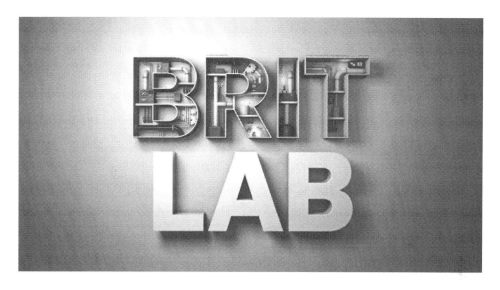

(Brit Lab, 2015)

Video discussing the invention, the effects, and the controversy surrounding LSD. Also, the video discusses the absence of overdoses from LSD and some of the potential implications to users' mental health.

Recreational use of LSD became popular during the 1960s in the United States and Western Europe, and, during this period, the use of the drug and advocacy of it became widespread (LSD, 2016). LSD became a symbol of the counterculture during this period, and the drug's influence can be seen in the music and art that were developed during this period. The promotion of the drug during the 1960s through the music and art of the period were widespread, and experimentation with the drug was common until the mid-1970s when information about the negative psychological effects was released to the general public. There have been periods in which revival of the drug has occurred since the 1960s, and the most notable of these was in the 1990s in the US and other regions throughout the world.

Chapter 2: Mental and Physiological Effects of LSD

Serotoninergic hallucinogens, which include LSD, psilocybin, and DMT, cause mainly visual and perceptual disturbances that resemble those observed in individuals developing the early signs of schizophrenia (Schmid et al., 2015). These hallucinogens result in altered information processing that is similar to those of individuals diagnosed with schizophrenia, which is measured by researchers through prepulse inhibition. The PPI measurements of LSD and other serotoninergic hallucinogens are similar to those observed in the early phases of the onset of schizophrenia. The effects of LSD begin thirty to sixty minutes after ingesting the drug, and the peak effects are generally felt around two hours after the drug is taken. LSD results in an alteration of users' waking consciousness, which includes hallucinations, synesthesia, and depersonalization. LSD typically does not produce high levels of anxiety for most users, and feelings of improved well-being, happiness, and trust of others are increased in environments in which sessions occur. The psychological effects of LSD use generally last between twelve and sixteen hours, but this is dependent on the amount of the drug taken and the level of tolerance users have to it. The effects of LSD are considered to last about as long as the duration of mescaline sessions and longer than psilocybin and DMT, which can last up to six hours for psilocybin and less than an hour for DMT.

The psychological and physiological effects of LSD differ from other serotoninergic hallucinogens, specifically the blissful state felt, ego dissolution, and visionary restructuralization (Schmid et al., 2015). In the aforementioned mention areas, LSD produces 30% higher ratings in comparison to psilocybin and 50% higher ratings than both DMT and ketamine. LSD has been found to produce less anxiety than psilocybin, but it has a higher amphetamine-like effect in comparison to the euphoria and empathy experienced from empathogens. Overall, LSD has similar visual and ego dissolution seen in the effects of psilocybin, and users report positive feelings and closeness to others, which are comparable to the effects of 3,4-methylenedioxy-methamphetamine or MDMA. Researchers attribute the empathogen-like effects of users LSD experiences to increased oxytocin levels, which is associated with the serotoninergic and oxytocinergic properties of the drug. MDMA has been found to produce weaker hallucinations in users in comparison to LSD, which is attributed to its 5-HT2A receptor stimulation. LSD, however, acts as a direct partial agonist to serotoninergic receptors and MDMA acts an indirect serotoninergic agonist through its release of serotonin through serotonin transporter sights in pre-synaptic neurons within the brain.

Serotonin Agonist

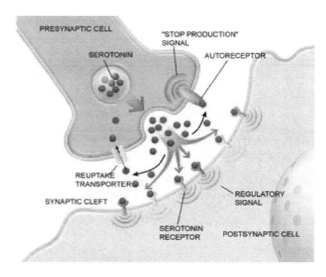

(Ghent University, 2016)

This image shows how serotonin receptor agonists work. LSD is a direct partial agonist, which means that it is a compound that activates receptors similar to serotonin in the brain.

Indirect Agonist

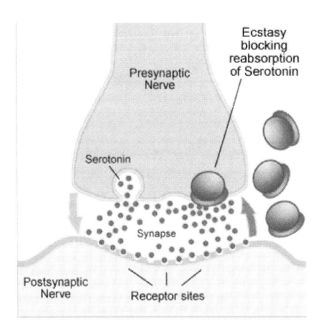

(Herballove, 2016)

Indirect agonists, like MDMA, enhance the action of neurotransmission, and they block the reuptake of serotonin. Therefore, the synapse becomes flooded with serotonin, which results in the effects that classify it as an empathogen.

The primary concerns in contemporary research regarding the use of serotoninergic hallucinogens are psychological rather than potential adverse physiological effects because a small number of users report moderate levels of anxiety in the initial stages of the onset of the drugs (Schmid et al., 2015). There have been a few cases of individuals reporting large amounts of anxiety when administered LSD in LSD-assisted psychotherapy research. This anxiety results from a fear of the power of the drug, feelings of lack of thought control, disembodiment, and depersonalization, which are common side effects associated with the use of the drug. Anxiety has been found to be present in both participants who have recreationally experienced serotoninergic hallucinogens and to new users. LSD disrupts the prepulse inhibition at a higher rate than other serotoninergic hallucinogens and exhibits similar levels to those found in schizophrenics. High PPI levels have only been found LSD and psilocybin use, but similar PPI levels have not been reported with research regarding the use of DMT or ayahuasca in humans.

Serotoninergic hallucinogens, like LSD, target the 5-HT2A receptor (Schmid et al., 2015). This is unregulated in individuals suffering from schizophrenia, and research has shown that there are genetic variations in the 5-HT2A receptor, which can lead to different levels of stimulation of the receptor site with different outcomes and varying PPI levels in participants. Sympathomimetic effects of LSD increase users' blood pressure, heart rates, and pupil sizes. These findings were reported in initial studies of the drug in the 1950s, and the cardiological effects of LSD are considered to be moderate in comparison to the effects seen in empathogens and stimulants. LSD use increases epinephrine levels in users similarly to those seen in MDMA, and the thermogenic response to LSD is considered to be weaker than MDMA but has resulted similarly in hyperthermic overdose in a few reported cases. Serotoninergic hallucinogens have also been found to increase circulating levels of cortisol and prolactin in plasma in humans, but these findings have not been found to be true in studies with laboratory animals and are considered to vary in humans in relation to the dosage of the drug administered. Although the use of LSD in laboratory settings in conjunction with psychotherapy has allowed researchers to investigate the psychological and physiological response to the drug, it is recognized that the psychological effects and risks associated with the drug greatly differ when used recreationally or by individuals with psychiatric disorders.

LSD's effects on perception and mood are similar to those found in MDMA, and it is these empathogenic properties that psychotherapists think may offer beneficial outcomes for the use of the drug in clinical settings as a result of the increased plasma oxytocin levels that follow ingestion of the drug (Schmid et al., 2015). LSD use does produce prepulse inhibition levels at rates seen in individuals suffering from schizophrenia, so it is possible that future studies involving the drug may assist in clinical assistance to those suffering from the disease. LSD is a powerful serotoninergic hallucinogen that has the ability to alter information processing and consciousness in humans because of its psychopharmacologic effects. It is clear that the drug has potential beneficial outcomes when used in clinical settings in conjunction with psychotherapy to treat a wide variety of psychological disorders. The positive effects of the drug in combination with the potential benefits should continue to be studied by researchers.

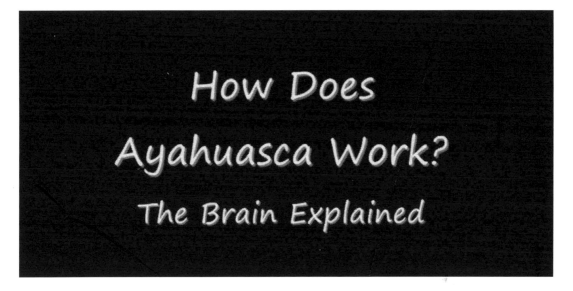

(Galactic Scholar Consciousness, 2013)

Video explaining how ayahuasca, a serotoninergic hallucinogen, affects the brain. This drug targets the 5-HT2A receptor similarly to LSD, but it has some differing psychological and physiological effects on users. The video discusses how the drug targets both similar and differing areas of the brain, which results in the differing effects.

Chapter 3: Hallucinogens

A hallucinogen is a drug that is synthesized or occurs naturally that produces psychological effects that can be associated with dreams, religious joy, or psychosis (Hallucinogen, 2016). These drugs change users' perceptions, thoughts, and feelings, and these changes result in both illusions and hallucinations. Hallucinogens increase users' sensory signals, but they typically result in a loss of control over what is experienced and felt. The most popular and most controversial hallucinogens are LSD, mescaline, psilocybin and psilocin, bufotenine, harmine, MDMA, phencyclidine, and tetrahydrocannabinol. LSD was originally extracted from ergot or Claviceps purpurea, which is a fungus found in rye and wheat. Mescaline is derived from the peyote cactus or lophophora williamsii, and it grows in the United States in the Southwest and parts of Mexico. Psilocybin and psilocin come from hundreds of mushrooms species from around the world, but two of the most common are psilocybe mexicana and stropharia cubensis, which are both found throughout North America. Bufotenine is isolated from the skin of a toad, and harmine is extracted from the seed coat of a plant found in the Middle East and throughout the Mediterranean. Both MDMA and phencyclidine are synthetic compounds created in laboratories, and tetrahydrocannabinol is the active ingredient found in marijuana, which is obtained from the flowers of female plants.

Hallucinogens have been used for thousands of years by native tribes prior to them being outlawed in Western societies, specifically by the Aztecs and, more recently, the Apache Tribe of the US (Hallucinogen, 2016). In 1918, the use of peyote for religious worship was legalized for the Native American Church following its adoption of Christianity. Scientists have been interested in hallucinogens for the last two centuries with the isolation of the active ingredient in peyote in the late nineteenth century, and the creation of LSD by Albert Hoffmann in Switzerland in the mid-twentieth century. The power of psilocybin's and psilocin's hallucinogenic effects were investigated by mycologist, Gordon Wasson, in the mid-twentieth century as well. Although scientists do not fully understand how hallucinogens affect the brain, it is believed that they act as an antagonist toward serotonin, which is an import biogenic amine for neurotransmission. Research on hallucinogens in conjunction with psychotherapy was used throughout the 1950s and 1960s, but the majority of research findings concluded that the side effects of these drugs were serious, which resulted in an end to most human experimentation and legal synthesis of the drugs.

Despite the findings from research studies in the mid-twentieth century, illicit experimentation has continued, and it has resulted in a subculture that endorsed hallucinogen use since (Hallucinogen, 2016). This subculture initially began in the Western United States, and it spread throughout North America to Europe and Australia. At the end of the twentieth century and into the twenty-first century, the use of MDMA and new substances, like phenethylamine and tryptamine, became more widespread and easy to manufacture because of information readily available online. It is clear that both synthetic and natural hallucinogens will be continued to be used by subcultures throughout the world despite government prohibition of them, and, as more individuals gain education regarding pharmacology and psychopharmacology, new and better hallucinogens will most likely be produced.

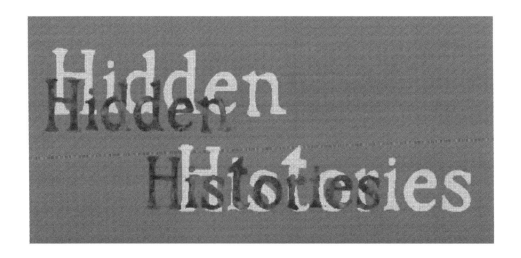

(Archaesoup Productions, 2011)

Video discussing the history of hallucinogens used by ancient cultures for religious purposes throughout the world. It is clear from the video that hallucinogens have been used throughout human history, and it can be concluded that they will be continued to be used by humans well into the future for cultural reasons.

Chapter 4: Reviving LSD Studies

The first intentional use of LSD was done by the creator of the drug, Albert Hofmann, in 1943 in which he ingested 250 micrograms in a laboratory setting prior to riding his bicycle home (Carhart-Harris et al., 2016). A detailed report of his experience that was written a few days following the session discusses his altered perception, fear, and paranoia as a result of the hallucinogen. His report describes the visual transformation of his neighbor, a disintegration of his environment, the suppression of his ego, and trepidation of going insane. He, however, disclosed that following the session he awoke the next morning feeling well and felt a sensation of renewed wellbeing. In his account, he discusses deriving pleasure from his breakfast and a walk through his garden in conjunction with an impression that the world around him was fresh and newly created.

LSD was first distributed by Sandoz Pharmaceuticals in 1948 for analytical psychotherapy research and experimental studies on mental disorders (Carhart-Harris et al., 2016). The rationale behind its use for analytical psychotherapy was that LSD could be used to elicit repressed memories and provide relaxation with individuals that have obsession disorders, and it could be used in experimental research investigations to model psychoses and understand the nature of the diseases. These two areas formed the basis for most research projects using the drug during the 1950s and 1960s, but many contemporary researchers believe that the psychopathology of the drug was not properly address during these decades of research prior to them ending. Contemporary researchers are attempting to address the paradox that LSD can be both a model and treatment for mental disorders, and modern research studies are attempting to address the underlying contradiction of hallucinogens, specifically LSD.

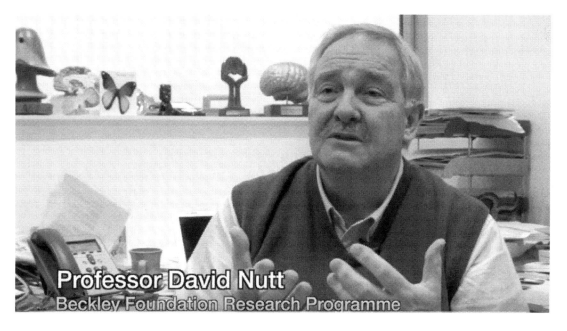

(Walacea, 2015)

Video discussing and promoting contemporary LSD research and studies regarding psychedelics, and the importance of the knowledge gained from the studies of the drug resulting from our lack of understanding about the pharmacodynamics of the drug.

Prior to the drug's cessation of clinical studies on humans due to political pressure in the 1960s, psychiatrists theorized in the early years of research that individuals suffering from schizophrenia possibly had an LSD-like schizotoxin in their brains, and, in the later years of initial LSD research, researchers focused more on the therapeutic applications of the drug in treating drug dependence and anxiety disorders (Carhart-Harris et al., 2016). At the end of human research using LSD in the 1960s because of government regulation, there was some reported success in the use of the drug in treating various mental disorders. LSD has not been studied in a laboratory environment on human subjects for nearly fifty years, but, since 2010, research studies have been permitted by ethics committees in some Western nations. Therefore, some new research studies have begun.

Clinical research using psychedelics, specifically LSD, began again in 2010, and the revival of studies has revealed the paradoxical nature of hallucinogens that was reported by scientists at the end of LSD research on humans in the 1960s (Carhart-Harris et al., 2016). From contemporary research, it is clear that the use of hallucinogens has different outcomes for different subjects, but, in a study using psilocybin, 80% of volunteers reported improved wellbeing following their session in conjunction with a follow-up to the study in which 65% of the individuals reported the same sense of comfort level more than a year after the experiment. Similar findings have been reported in other studies using psilocybin in which the drug has been used in conjunction with psychotherapy to treat addiction, obsessive-compulsive disorder, and anxiety disorders. Most of the studies report that individuals experience some fear and psychological discomfort during their sessions, but the therapeutic benefits have far outweighed these negative aspects of the sessions and have been enduring. Thus, it can be concluded that the use of hallucinogens has had therapeutic success in clinical settings in conjunction with psychotherapy in the twenty-first century, and the revival of the research that was discontinued by Western governments in the 1960s has proven to be beneficial to medical science.

Western governments ended psychedelic research because of case reports regarding recreational users committing suicide and having mental health problems (Carhart-Harris et al., 2016). Contemporary research, however, has shown that cases leading to negative outcomes as a result of the recreational use of psychedelics are rare, and there have been very few case reports regarding negative outcomes of the use of psychedelics in clinical settings. The evidence collected in the twenty-first century regarding the recreational use of psychedelics has been found to contradict government reports released in the 1960s in relation to the negative outcomes of their use, and population studies of the recreational use of the drug have shown that it actually decreases suicidal thoughts and psychological distress among recreational users. Most importantly there has been almost no evidence that the use of psychedelics has led to mental health problems, and large meta-analyses of users of the drugs have reported that less than .1% of users experience negative outcomes following their use.

In contemporary research studies using LSD, psychotomimetic states can be considered to be high in comparison to studies on sleep deprivation, MDMA, psilocybin, ketamine, and tetrahydrocannabinol (Carhart-Harris et al., 2016). Volunteers in contemporary research studies have shown psychotic behavior and thinking, such as delusions and paranoia, during LSD sessions. Overall, most participants have reported positive experiences and moods during sessions, which is consistent with the research findings and paradoxical nature of the drug that were reported in the 1960s prior to the cessation of research being permitted using human participants and the drug. For most participants, reports of optimism and openness increase in the weeks following LSD sessions in comparison to control groups, and there are typically no increased reports in psychotic symptoms following use of the drug, which are consistent with research studies from the 1960s on LSD and other contemporary studies on hallucinogens. In general, it can be concluded that the use of psychedelics, like LSD, lead to positive outcomes in relation to mood and mental health in both LSD research and recreational use, which has also been a consistent finding in relation to the use of LSD and other hallucinogens in research on treating psychiatric disorders.

Optimism and openness increase with psychedelic use, specifically with LSD, in the vast majority of users, and research studies involving human trials with LSD use in the twenty-first century have concluded that these traits are reliable in both short-term and long-term self-reports following laboratory testing (Carhart-Harris et al., 2016). Researchers have concluded from the data of the studies conducted in the 1960s and studies with more contemporary designs that the use of LSD can be used to preserve and better the mental health of individuals. They have also found that the use of psychedelics, including LSD, can be useful in treating individuals with mental disorders, and, in general, there is strong evidence that LSD and other psychedelic drugs can be used to treat individuals with mood disorders and to improve socio-economic outcomes of patients with a range of therapeutic needs. It is clear that there a paradoxical effects to the use of psychedelics in both laboratory and recreational settings, and this fact contributed to the ban on the sale, manufacturing, and testing of the drug in Western nations. The acute effects that lead to fear and paranoia in the short-term for some patients under the influence of LSD in conjunction with psychotherapy in laboratory settings are clearly paradoxical, but the long-term effects of the drug far outweigh the acute

effects and are more clinically relevant.

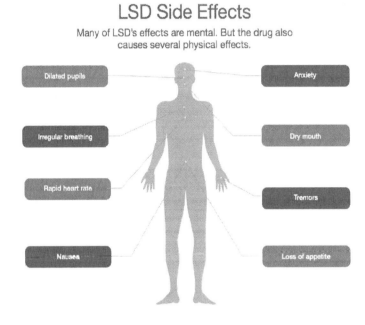

(Williams, 2015)

This image shows the physical effects of LSD, but research has uncovered the paradoxical nature of the drug, which causes fear and paranoia in some users. The physiological and short-term mental effects are far surpassed by the therapeutic benefits the drug offers for a wide-variety of mental disorders, and the long-term outcomes associated with its use.

Chapter 5: Neural Activity and Hallucinations

The neural mechanisms that are responsible for hallucinations are not well-understood by neurologists, and the underlying reason for this is because hallucinations occur with a great deal of content and happen under a variety of conditions (Iaria et al., 2010). Hallucinations occur as a result of "hypnagogic states and visual sensory deprivation in healthy subjects, visual loss in brain damaged patients, neurologic conditions", disease, psychiatric conditions, and withdrawal states from substance abuse (Iaria et al., 2010, p. 106). In each of the former conditions, hallucinations can occur simultaneously between objects, people, and actions performed in both familiar and unfamiliar environments, which makes it difficult to understand the neural mechanisms related to perceptions caused by hallucinations.

Research into both auditory and visual hallucinations has allowed investigation into what is happening in the brain when individuals undergo these phenomena, and the use of neuroimaging techniques over the last three decades has allowed scientists to begin to understand what is occurring in the human brain with the use of positron emission tomography and functional magnetic resonance imaging when people hallucinate (Allen et at. 2008). Based on the findings from contemporary research regarding hallucinations using PET and fMRI brain scans, there is a network of brain areas involved in both auditory and visual hallucinations, and it is clear that several alterations to activation and functional connectivity between a network of regions of the brain are integral to the process of both auditory and visual hallucinations as it pertains to the process of conscious perception. For auditory hallucinations, there is increased activation of the left posterior superior temporal gyrus, and, for visual hallucinations, there is hyperactivation of the secondary sensory cortex. In both auditory and visual hallucinations, there is also activation of the primary auditory cortex and primary perceptual cortex, which are considered to be responsible for processing low-level aspects of perception. There is a great deal of information non-sensory regions of the brain in a distributed network of cortical and subcortical regions involved in the hallucinatory process. In comparison to the non-hallucinating brain, a hallucinating brain has reduced gray matter volumes in the temporal cortex, increased activation in the subcortical centers, and less control in the dorsolateral prefrontal cortex. There is irregular activation from the ventral and dorsal regions of the anterior cingulate cortex, supplementary motor area, and cerebellum, which are involved in monitoring processes within the brain. Dysfunction of these brain areas apply to both auditory and visual hallucinations, and it accounts for the emotions experienced, feeling of externality, and lack of will that accompany individuals experiences. It is believed for auditory hallucinations that are seen in psychotic illnesses that they are caused as a result of altered activation of the inferior frontal gyrus and anterior cingulate, which are the speech production areas and the language reception areas of the brain.

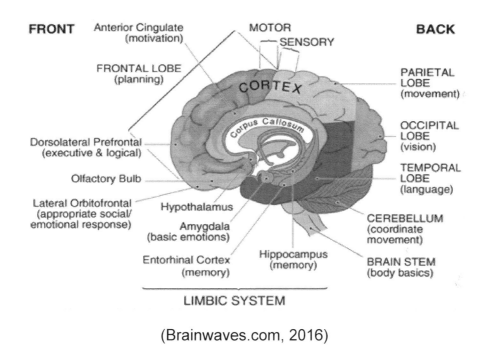

(Brainwaves.com, 2016)

Image depicting the different parts of the brain. It is believed that auditory hallucinations are a result of altered activation in inferior frontal gyrus and anterior cingulate.

The two neurotransmitters that are important to visual hallucinations are serotonin and acetylcholine, and they are concentrated in the visual thalamic nuclei and visual cortex (Manford & Andermann, 1998). Visual hallucinations that are experienced by individuals are a result of cholinergic-serotonergic interactions in either the visual thalamus or the visual cortex. Hallucinations caused by LSD and mescaline target serotonin receptors concentrated in the cerebral cortex, and serotonergic neurons are believed to cause visual hallucinations as a result of the modulatory effect of the sensory pathways and cortical responses, which results in a disturbance to the visual pathway and brainstem. Visual hallucinations, caused from drug use or pathologies, affect the brain similarly in that they alter the cortico-cortical inputs and serotonergic inputs, which change the normal regulation of processes in the visual association cortex and reticular activating system in the brain.

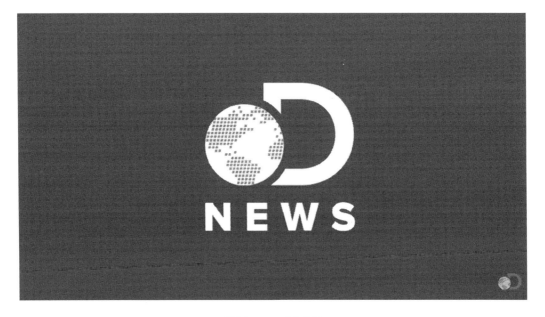

(DNews, 2015)

Video discussing brain activity during both auditory and visual hallucinations that result from both psychosis and drug use.

Chapter 6: LSD, Visual Hallucinations, and Brain Function

LSD is both a prototypical and unique psychedelic drug because it has had a large impact on science, the arts, and society following its discovery, which has resulted from its widespread use and the life-changing experiences that users have had (Carthart-Harris et al., 2016). Following contemporary studies of the drug, researchers have shown that the drug has typical conscious-altering effects that are seen in other hallucinogens in relation to blood flow, neural activity, and communication patterns through neuroimaging techniques. The implications for neurobiology and psychology are great because new psychological and physiological information is being uncovered as a result of contemporary studies of the drug, which extend the research on the potential therapeutic benefits of the drug that were being investigated by researchers prior to a ban on LSD research with humans in the mid-1960s. The LSD state results in increased cerebral blood flow to the visual cortex, resting state functional connectivity, and decreased alpha power, which can be used to predict the magnitude of visual hallucinations experienced by users. Changes in users' consciousness and the subsequent ego-dissolution following the ingestion of LSD results from decreased default-mode network, parahippocampal retrosplenial cortex resting state functional connectivity, and delta and alpha power released. There is a strong relationship between primary visual cortex resting state functional connectivity and decreased alpha power in the brain under the influence of LSD, specifically the relationship between visual hallucinations experienced on the drug and the decreased alpha power to the occipital sensors. The discovery of this relationship is novel, and the finding shows that there is a greater proportion of the brain contributing to visual processing when in an LSD state than under normal conditions.

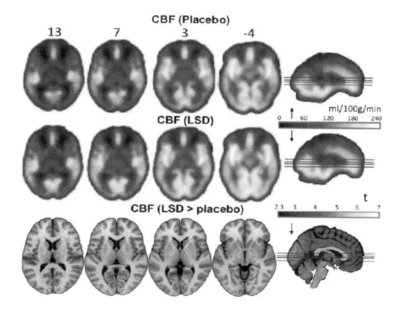

(Carthart-Harris et al., 2016, p. 4854)

This image shows the cerebral blood flow of a normal brain and a brain on LSD. The image on the bottom shows the difference of the increased blood flow when comparing a brain on LSD to a normal brain.

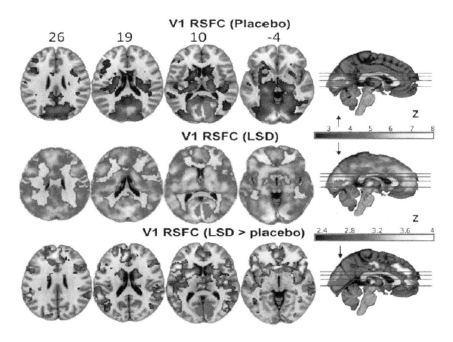

(Carthart-Harris et al., 2016, p. 4855)

This image shows the difference between the primary visual cortex resting state functional connectivity of a normal brain and a brain on LSD. The image on the bottom shows the difference of the increased blood flow when comparing a brain on LSD to a normal brain.

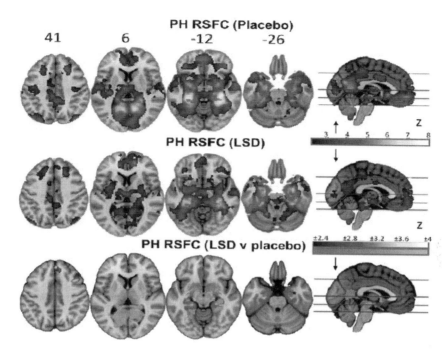

(Carthart-Harris et al., 2016, p. 4855)

This image shows parahippocampal resting state functional connectivity between a normal brain and a brain on LSD. The image on the bottom shows the difference of the increased blood flow when comparing a normal brain to a brain on LSD. This effect is believed to contribute to the ego-dissolution that is experienced by users while in an LSD state.

It is clear that psychedelics, like LSD, impair and reduce the stability of brain networks during a psychedelic state in conjunction with increasing the integration of neural networks within the brain (Carthart-Harris et al., 2016). There are some specific physiological effects on the brain that occur when under the influence of psychedelic drugs, specifically disordered cortical activity. The visual hallucinations that are experienced while using psychedelics are a result of the increased primary visual cortex resting state functional connectivity, and the level of disassociation of the parahippocampal retrosplenial cortex relates to the magnitude of ego dissolution and the deep thought that occurs in a psychedelic state. It is clear that the neurobiology of psychedelic hallucinations and the ego-dissolution resulting from LSD states can better inform us regarding visual processing and the importance of areas of the brain in the maintenance of individuals' concepts of self. Contemporary research has offered new evidence of the potential for psychedelic drugs to be used for therapy, and, as we continue to understand better how these drugs work in the brain, neurobiologists and psychotherapists may be able to use psychedelic drugs in the future to treat embed core pathological behaviors resulting from psychiatric disorders by dismantling patterns of activity.

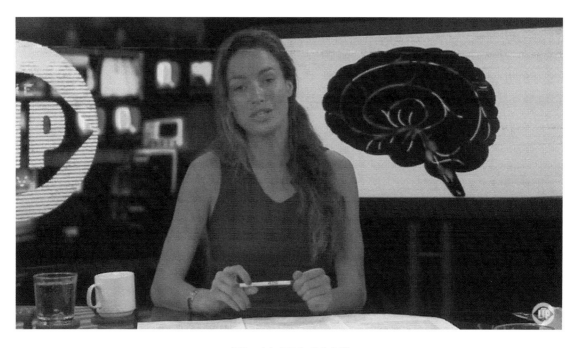

(TheLipTV, 2016)

Video discussing what new research has revealed regarding LSD and the implications of it for scientific understanding regarding the brain and therapy for individuals suffering from psychiatric disorders.

Chapter 7: Behavioral Pharmacology of LSD State

The pharmacological action of LSD's effects on the brain is not fully understood, but the 5-HT and the 5-HT2A receptors are believed to play a large role in mediating the effects of hallucinogens (Schindler et al., 2012). The two major classes of hallucinogens can be divided into two categories: phenethylamines and tryptamines. An example of a drug with phenethylamine would be mescaline, and an example of a drug with tryptamine would be LSD. Hallucinogens are considered to have significant value by researchers because they have helped to model psychosis, and they have improved scientific understanding of cognition and perception in humans. The psychological effects of hallucinogens, like LSD, are now considered essential for some types of therapy, but the paradoxical nature, strength of the drugs, and potential psychosis will ultimately limit their widespread use for therapy with patients with mental disorders. There are some advantages to using hallucinogens in comparison to both licit and illicit drugs because they are not addictive and, for most users, lead to positive and beneficial outcomes when used in the correct environment, under the correct dosage, and with the correct psychotherapy.

In laboratory studies with mice, head twitches are used to measure the dose and outcomes related to hallucinogens that are used for both therapy and recreation by humans (Schindler et al., 2012). Research regarding the effects of hallucinogens in laboratory animals has shown scientists the level of involvement of serotonin receptors in hallucinogenic states because the same behavioral effects are not observed when serotonin agonists are used in conjunction with the drugs. Serotonergic antagonists, like cyproheptadine, methysergide, and bromo-LSD, block head twitches in mice and other rodents, and this is believed to be a result of them not affecting the 5-HT2A receptor similarly to both phenethylamines and tryptamines. The evidence from serotonergic antagonists suggests that the 5-HT2A receptor is necessary for hallucinogenic states and subsequent effects felt by humans while using the drugs. Evidence regarding the targeting of serotonin receptors and its effects varies between species, and it is believed to be a result of the complexity or lack thereof in various species. For example, the 5-HT2C was found to result in head twitches in mice but not in rats. This evidence has not been found for any rodent species regarding the injection of hallucinogens in the frontal cortex, which elicits head twitches as a result of the brain region having a large number of 5-HT2A receptors in nearly all rodent species. Because of the number of 5-HT2A receptors in the frontocortical area of the brain, it is considered an important area of investigation in analyzing the effects of hallucinogens and the role of serotonin receptors.

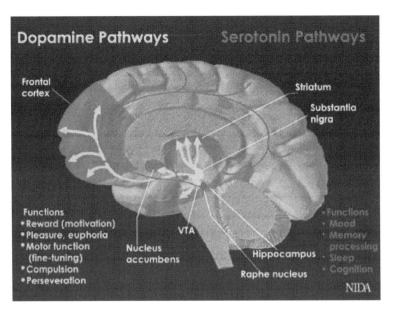

(NIDA, 2016)

This image shows the dopamine and serotonin pathways in conjunction with the prefrontal cortex, which plays an important role in bringing about the LSD state.

The dopaminergic system is thought by researchers to play a significant role in human psychosis, which is a state that hallucinogens imitate (Schindler et al., 2012). Hallucinogens, however, differ in their dopaminergic pharmacologic action. A good example would be how LSD binds with dopamine receptors in the human brain but 2,5-dimethoxy-4-iodoamphetamine does not. The investigation of dopaminergic receptors has resulted in the improved scientific understanding of the pharmacology and subsequent behaviors that result from hallucinogens, and it has offered new insights into the brain mechanisms involved in human consciousness and psychosis. Dopamine receptor antagonists have shown to block twitches in rodents under the influence of DOI, which has shown that the

hallucinogenic effects resulting from DOI ingestion are dependent on interaction

with receptors in the dopaminergic system.

Cl—H

(Novachem, 2015)

This image shows the chemical structure of 2,5-dimethoxy-4-iodoamphetamine or
DOI, which are typically used as a substitute for amphetamines. DOI is a
psychedelic drug that has similar effects to LSD, but the effects are considered to
be longer, resulting in different hallucinogenic experiences in combination with
feeling more energetic.

Both LSD and DOI cause head twitches in rodents in laboratory settings

through 5-HT2A receptor activation (Schindler et al., 2012). This suggests that

both LSD and DOI pharmacologic action causing in similar behavior and effects are a result of similar serotonin pathways affected in the brain, specifically the frontocortical area of the brain. The dopaminergic system is strongly linked to human consciousness, and research has shown that dopamine regulation is strongly tied to psychotic disease in humans, which is a condition that arises in most hallucinogenic experiences. LSD targets dopamine receptors, and it is believed to play central a role in the LSD state. Activation of dopamine receptors has been shown to cause head twitches in rodents when injected with LSD, and there is a lack of head twitching in conditions in which dopamine antagonists are used. Therefore, researchers have concluded that dopamine receptors are important in LSD pharmacological action. LSD has a stronger effect on dopamine receptors in the frontal cortex in comparison with other hallucinogens, but the relationship between both the 5-HT2A and D1 receptors are considered to play both a direct and indirect role in all hallucinogenic experiences, especially in humans. Although the importance of the dopamine receptors for DOI pharmacologic action is less than LSD, it still plays an indirect role in the drug's effects. The relationship between both serotonin and dopamine receptors and pathways play a central role in the hallucinogenic experience in humans. It is clear that each hallucinogen is unique in its pharmacology but similar areas of the brain are targeted, which result in varying hallucinogenic experiences depending on which drug is used. The effects of hallucinogens are similar and uniquely distinct in relation to their use by humans, and it is clear that there is a lot that is not fully understood in regards to hallucinogenic compounds because of their powerful effects resulting in long-lasting psychological changes. Thus, it can be concluded that the interactions of hallucinogens with individuals' genetic makeup and neurocircuitry are unique in their psychological effects and not fully understood by scientists. Each hallucinogen may target similar pathways to others, but the subtle difference in the receptors that are targeted and relied upon ultimately lead to different hallucinogenic experience and behavioral effects felt by users.

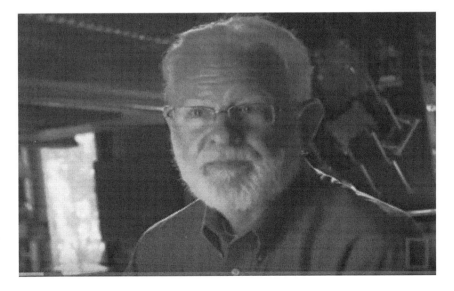

(Intergalatic, 2010)

Video discussing the effects of LSD in rodent experiments. It also discusses the implications of the drug's use and subsequent behavior, and the possible benefits of studying the effects of the drug in treating schizophrenia in humans.

Chapter 8: LSD Psychotherapy

Oral doses of more than one hundred micrograms of LSD results in users cause psychosensory changes that include increased sensory perception, illusionary changes of objects in their environments, synesthesia, and enhanced mental imagery (Gasser et al., 2014). Users' thoughts are accelerated and broadened in scope, and they usually result in new interpretations of emotions, relationships, and objects in environments. Emotions are usually aroused as a result of the underlying changes in users' psychological states in conjunction with hypermnesia and enhanced mental processing. The general state of users' consciousness has been compared to a daydream with increased emotion and inner stimuli in combination with weakened ego identification. Many researchers believe that LSD has the ability to amplify consciousness in users, and, as a result of the effects that last from six to nine hours, it is believed that LSD can support and enhance psychotherapeutic processing in users. The effects of LSD on the brain are complex and not fully understood, but it is agreed by neurologists that it has diverse influence over neurotransmitters within the brain, specifically through the serotonin receptors: 5-HT2A, 5-HT2C, and 5-HT1A.

The use of psychotherapy with psychedelic drugs began in the 1950s, and psychotherapists typically used the psycholytic method or the psychedelic method

(Gasser et al., 2014). The psycholytic method used lower doses with frequent psychotherapeutic sessions, and the psychedelic method used higher doses with fewer sessions. The goal of the psychedelic method was to induce moments of mystical experience and catharsis to enable patients to work through difficult feelings and situations in their lives to assist in reducing anxiety and depression regarding them. A study in 1963 found that the use of LSD with counseling was able to assist in reducing anxiety, depression, and pain in advanced-stage cancer patients, which was replicated in larger studies with the same results. LSD psychotherapy in the 1960s with terminally ill patients typically used the psychedelic method to assist in reducing anxiety, depression, and pain surrounding their diseases.

Research using LSD in conjunction with psychotherapy was done throughout the United States and Europe until 1966 when it became illegal as a result of increased non-medical use of the drug (Gasser et al., 2014). There was some research conducted using LSD in Germany, the Netherlands, and Czechoslovakia in the 1970s and, later, in Switzerland 1980s and 1990s. In 2011, the US and other Western governments began to permit research using LSD with human participants again, and the research findings with the use of LSD in treating individuals with terminal illness related anxiety and depression have been positive.

Group comparisons between participants who received a placebo and participants who received two hundred micrograms of LSD showed that there were no severe adverse effects to individuals who were administered the drug, and participants who received LSD-assisted psychotherapy showed reduced anxiety regarding their terminal illnesses in two sessions in comparison with participants who received placebos.

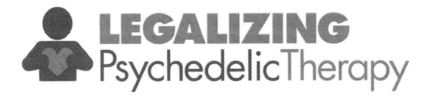

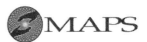

(Multidisciplinary Association for Psychedelic Therapy, 2014)

Video discussing the benefits for psychedelic-assisted psychotherapy and the need for continued research with the use of psychedelics in treating depression, anxiety, and PTSD.

Antidepressant, Anxiolytic, and Addiction Treatment with Serotoninergic Hallucinogens

The pharmacological treatments for mood and anxiety disorders for drug dependence that are presently used in contemporary medicine have shown little efficacy (Santos et al., 2016). Studies using LSD, psilocybin, and ayahuasca on animals in laboratory settings show that serotoninergic hallucinogens have antidepressive, anxiolytic, and antiaddictive properties that can benefit individuals suffering from drug dependence. LSD, psilocybin, and ayahuasca have beneficial effects in treating individuals that are showing resistance to traditional Western medicine and psychotherapy, psychological problems resulting from life-threatening diseases, and addiction to both licit and illicit substances. Serotoninergic hallucinogens are useful drugs in treating the aforementioned conditions, especially in situations in which patients that have shown treatment resistance to traditional methods. Serotoninergic hallucinogens also have the potential to increase scientific understanding regarding psychiatric disorders and may help researchers develop novel therapeutic remedies.

Serotoninergic hallucinogens not only have antidepressive, anxiolytic, and antiaddictive properties, but they also have low toxicity and are considered to be relatively safe when administered and used in supervised, controlled environments (Santos et al., 2016). Serotoninergic hallucinogens, like LSD and psilocybin, are less pharmacologically toxic and physiologically less harmful than the majority of both legal and illegal drugs. The mechanisms of action responsible for the benefits resulting from the use of serotoninergic hallucinogens in therapeutic settings are not fully understood by researchers, but it is clear that multiple studies of these substances over the last sixty-five years has resulted in conclusive evidence that these drugs have the ability to offer therapeutic benefits to patients, especially those showing resistance to traditional depression, anxiety, and addiction treatments. It is believed by researchers that the therapeutic effects of serotoninergic hallucinogens result from the drugs targeting of serotonin receptors, which has been shown to be altered in post-mortem samples of individuals who suffered from depressive disorders brains. This suggests that the 5-HT1A, 5-HT2A, and 5-HT2C receptors are involved in emotional processing in individuals, and this has been confirmed in laboratory experiments on animals. Clinical studies involving animals have shown that the 5-HT1A receptor has both anxiolytic and antidepressive properties, and the 5-HT2A and 5-HT2C receptors are involved in both anxiety and depression-related behavior. It is also believed that the therapeutic action of the drugs results from the activation of the frontocortical glutamate networks by the 5-HT2A receptor, which increases the expression of neurotrophic factors that increase neuroplasticity and neurogenesis in the brain.

Depression is associated with deficient neurogenesis and neurotrophic activity in patients, and they have been shown to normalize after treatment in patients.

The agonism produced by serotoninergic hallucinogens is thought to produce beneficial anti-inflammation effects due to their targeting of the 5-HT2A receptor (Santos et al., 2016). Research has shown that inflammatory cytokines are associated with depressive disorders and that these become normalized through antidepressant therapies. It is believed that this is a result of the agonism of the 5-HT2A receptor, which modulates the body's immune system. Both LSD and 2,5-dimethoxy-4-iodoamphetamine are 5-HT2A receptor agonists and have shown to produced anti-inflammatory effects in laboratory animals through blocking pro-inflammatory cell adhesion. Neural oxidative stress and the resulting neuroinflammation are associated with psychiatric disorders, and monoamine oxidase inhibitors used to treat depression stop harmine and harmaline inhibition, which has antioxidant and neuroprotective effects.

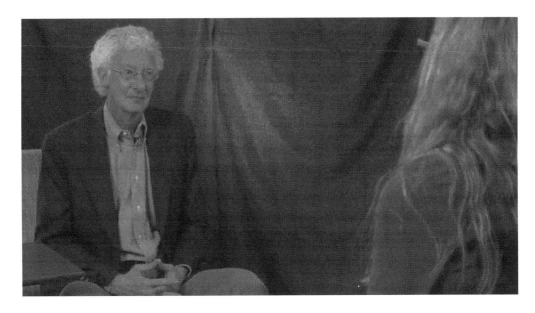

(Udacity, 2015)

Video discussing some of the potential negative side effects of serotoninergic hallucinogens and their potential to exacerbate underlying psychiatric conditions.

It is believed that the other aspects of modulation caused by serotoninergic hallucinogens, other than the targeting of the 5-HT1A, 5-HT2A, and 5-HT2C receptors, are involved in MAO inhibition, which results in decreased neuroinflammation and increased therapeutic action (Santos et al., 2016). The antiaddictive properties of serotoninergic hallucinogens are thought to be related to the dopaminergic system through indirect stimulation of dopaminergic pathways through 5-HT2A receptor activation. Research has shown that serotoninergic hallucinogens indirectly increase the release of dopamine in the ventral striatum in humans. Other research on laboratory animals has shown that the MAO inhibition of harmine and harmaline result in the antiaddictive properties through the "imidazoline, glutamate, and dopamine pathways" in the brain (Santos et al., 2016, p. 203).

Contemporary neuroimaging studies involving human participants have shown that the mood-enhancing properties of serotoninergic hallucinogens are related to modifications in brain activity in the amygdala and anterior cingulate cortex (Santos et al., 2016). These brain regions are involved in emotional processing, introspection, and other internally focused functions. Serotoninergic hallucinogens cause reduced amygdala reactivity and increased activity in the default mode network in the brain, which has been associated with positive mood and intensification of the important depressive symptoms causing rumination. Early research into serotoninergic hallucinogens has shown that these drugs have therapeutic properties as a result of their effects on users' perceptual activity, emotional response, and thought processes, which have been confirmed by more contemporary research that has included further investigation into the pharmacologic action of these drugs with neuroimaging studies. The psychological experiences and physiological effects of these drugs create an opportunity in which individuals can change unhealthy thoughts, feelings, and behaviors in therapeutic environments. Serotoninergic hallucinogens create an altered state of consciousness that allows individuals to interrupt normative repetitive, rigid, and pathological patterns, which can lead to negative thoughts, anxiety, and mood disorders. Many of these disorders are self-medicated by individuals, and this leads to both licit and illicit drug addictions. Serotoninergic hallucinogens assist individuals in developing mental flexibility that leads to changes in perspectives, values, and behavior. Some researchers believe that the peak experience resulting from the effects of serotoninergic hallucinogens elicits religious and mystical feelings that are associated with psychological benefits. Acute administration of serotoninergic hallucinogens has been shown in research studies to induce highly meaningful experiences to individuals that result in personally significant experiences and contribute to sustained positive "attitudes, mood, personality, and behavior" in users (Santos et al., 2016, p. 204). These mystical and religious associations have also found to assist in the cessation of both licit and illicit drug use and their dependence. Some researchers have associated the mental state produced by serotoninergic hallucinogens as inverse post-traumatic stress disorder in which the highly positive experiences associated with using the drugs lead to lasting beneficial mood and behavioral changes.

It is clear that serotoninergic hallucinogens have beneficial effects in treating mood, anxiety, and dependence disorders, especially in therapeutically assisting patients that are showing standard treatment-resistance (Santos et al., 2016). Research has shown that standard treatments for depression, anxiety, and drug dependence have limited efficacy and can often produce adverse reactions that result in limited or discontinued treatment. Serotoninergic hallucinogens administered in a controlled setting in conjunction with psychotherapeutic techniques have the potential to assist treatment-resistant patients with depression, anxiety, and addiction. The beneficial properties of serotoninergic hallucinogens are mediated by the agonist action on the 5-HT1A, 5-HT2A, and 5-HT2C receptors, which are involved "in emotional processing, regulation of neurotrophic factors, anti-inflammatory actions, and modulation of frontal and medial brain structures" (Santos et al., 2016, p. 205). There are other mechanisms of action, which are not related to serotoninergic receptors, which also mediate these therapeutic effects.

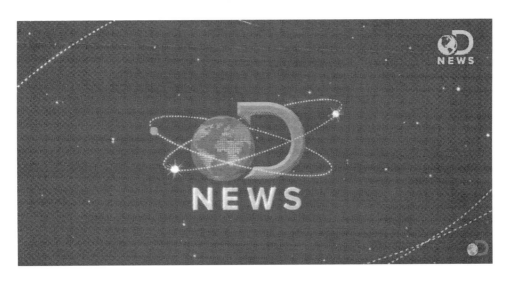

(DNews, 2014)

Video discussing how serotoninergic hallucinogens affect users psychologically and physiologically. It discusses some of the theories surrounding the drugs and new information regarding the pharmacologic action of the drugs.

Chapter 9: Bromo-LSD

Cluster headaches are series of short but extremely painful headaches that can afflict individuals on daily, weekly, or monthly (WebMD, 2016). They have a tendency to be seasonal in nature, and individuals that suffer from the condition have reported that they generally get them at the same time annually. Often, people suffering from the condition are unaware that they suffer from cluster headaches, and they mistake them for allergies or just general stress. Researchers are unaware of what causes cluster headaches, but they do know that nerves, specifically in the facial region, are involved. Cluster headaches are more severe than migraines, but they are shorter in duration. These headaches are more common in males than in females, and they affect less than one in a thousand individuals. People suffering from them typically start to get them before the age of thirty, and they sometimes go into remission or disappear completely.

Cluster headaches are categorized by severe orbital and periorbital pain, and they are categorized as either chronic or episodic (Karst et al., 2010). Individuals that suffer from cluster headaches use oxygen and sumatriptan, and they are also prescribed verapamil, lithium, corticosteroids, and other neuromodulators to help suppress attacks during periods that they are experienced. In general, standard treatments are reported to have limited efficacy or to be totally ineffective, and surgical treatment is an option, which results in deep brain or occipital nerve stimulation. There can be serious complications from these surgeries, which can result in nerve damage, brain damage, and, in some instances, death.

Due to the lack of efficacy of the drugs prescribe and the potential complications resulting from surgery, individuals suffering from cluster headaches have turned to obtaining and using serotoninergic hallucinogens illicitly to gain relief from this condition (Karst et al., 2010). Many of the individuals would use the serotoninergic hallucinogens, despite the unwanted effects that occur while using the drug, because the compounds offer relief that is far superior to legal alternatives. Researchers wanted to find an alternative for individuals suffering from cluster headaches in which they could get the benefits serotoninergic hallucinogens without the hallucinations, synesthesia, and depersonalization associated with LSD. The hallucinogenic effects of LSD are completely lost when "the double bond in the D ring is saturated" and substituted with R2 (Karst et al., 2010, p. 1140).

(Royal Society of Chemistry, 2015)

Image depicting the structure of 2-Bromo-LSD, which is a non-psychedelic derivative of LSD used in the treatment of cluster headaches.

Past studies using 2-Bromo-LSD have concluded that it is non-toxic and non-hallucinogenic, and it is only associated with mild side effects similarly to that of LSD because it binds to many of the same receptor sites (Karst et al., 2010). There have been no behavioral or psychological side effects associated with the use of 2-Bromo-LSD, and it has conclusively been shown to not alter psychosis. Research related to the use of 2-Bromo-LSD has shown that using the drug can break cluster headache cycles and can decrease the frequency and intensily of attacks. It has also shown to change cluster headaches from the chronic to the episodic form, and it has conclusively resulted in extending the remission of the onset of cluster headache attacks in many patients suffering from the disease. It is clear from the illicit use serotoninergic hallucinogens by many individuals that suffer from cluster headaches that the mechanism of action of the drugs offer relief to the condition, but it is combined with the unwanted side effects typically associated with the use of serotoninergic hallucinogens. The use of 2-Bromo-LSD offers an alternative to treating cluster headaches that is both non-toxic and non-hallucinogenic, which has shown beneficial outcomes for individuals that are suffering from cluster headaches in breaking the cluster headache cycles and decreasing the frequency and intensity of the attacks. The ergotamines, which include LSD, 2-Bromo-LSD, dihydroergotamine, and methysergide, have positive effects on individuals suffering from cluster headaches "through serotonin-receptor, mediated vasoconstriction" (Karst et al., 2010, p. 1141). In relation to the lack of efficacy of standard treatments for cluster headaches and in conjunction with the positive research findings regarding the use of serotoninergic hallucinogens and 2-Bromo-LSD in treating them, their use in treating cluster headaches and other related disease, especially with 2-Bromo-LSD, must be given serious consideration by the medical community. There is clear evidence that serotoninergic hallucinogens and 2-Bromo-LSD reduce the pain and cycle of cluster headache attacks and can extend the cycle of remission of them, which is not possible with the current treatments being used for the disease today.

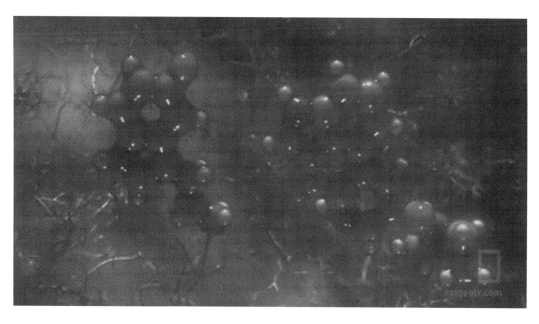

(Intergalactic, 2010)

Video discussing cluster headaches and the potential role that 2-Bromo-LSD could hold in assisting individuals that are afflicted with the disease.

Chapter 10: LSD, Interrogation, and Suggestibility

Following the discovery of LSD, the drug was investigated heavily by researchers as a psychotomimetic and tool to assist psychotherapists in treating patients with mental disorders (Carhart-Harris et al., 2015). It was also investigated in the 1960s, as a result of Cold War pressure, in a search to find new methods to enhance interrogation techniques and behavioral control. A program call MK-ULTRA was ordered by the United States Government to explore the potential of LSD to control individuals' minds and behavior. It was believed that the use of LSD could lead to increased suggestibility in individuals and increase their responsiveness to suggestions. Suggestions can lead to alterations of individuals' consciousness, and they can target individuals' perceptions, sensations, cognition, emotions, and behavior. Typically, a drug's level of suggestibility is measured by behavioral performance, and a classic response to suggestion would lead to an involuntary behavioral outcome in a participant. Suggestibility and the use of drugs allow individuals to respond involuntarily, and automatic responses have been demonstrated to be overcome as a result.

There were findings of increased suggestibility with the use of LSD in conjunction with psychotherapy and other research done by the MK-ULTRA Program in the 1950s and 1960s (Carhart-Harris et al., 2015). LSD's efficacy for suggestibility in combination with psychotherapy was revealed in the 1960s prior to its ban in 1966 throughout the world. LSD's efficacy for mind and behavioral control was never revealed through research by the MK-ULTRA Program, but the power of suggestibility in conjunction with psychotherapy was revealed in early studies of the drug. It is believed in contemporary research on LSD that suggestibility has played an important role in the efficacy of the drug in treating depression, anxiety, and addiction. Due to the power of LSD as a serotoninergic hallucinogen, there is concern that the efficacy of the drug in conjunction with its power of suggestibility can have both positive and negative implications for individuals under the influence. The power of the drug has the potential exploitation by therapists to implant false memories or beliefs in individuals undergoing LSD-assisted psychotherapy must be recognized and considered.

LSD targets many different neurotransmitter receptors, but it is believed that the main psychedelic effects associated with the use of the drug result from stimulation of 5-HT2A receptor (Carhart-Harris et al., 2015). Most serotoninergic hallucinogens have an affinity for the 5-HT2A receptor, which has been shown in research studies with the use of 5-HT2A agonists and serotoninergic hallucinogens. LSD has an especially high association with the 5-HT2A receptor and doses as low as twenty micrograms can produce psychedelic effects in humans. There have been findings that 5-HT2A signaling has been linked to increased cognitive flexibility, associative learning, and neural plasticity. This has serious implications in relation to the potential of the drug to be used for suggestibility because heightened neural plasticity is a prerequisite of it. The neural plasticity created as a result of the use of LSD can be exploited therapeutically for behavioral interventions in relation to addiction in which psychotherapy seeks "to extinguish reinforced behavior patterns" and "instate healthier ones" (Carhart-Harris et al., 2015, p. 791).

Neuroimaging studies with serotoninergic hallucinogens have shown decreased brain network integrity and increased network flexibility, and it is believed that this increases the suggestibility of individuals under the influence of the hallucinogenic drugs because of the suspension of reality testing in psychedelic states (Carhart-Harris et al., 2015). This acute drug state results in individuals feeling less assured regarding their beliefs, so they are increasingly receptive to external direction or suggestibility. Individuals, who are more trait conscientious, have been found to be highly suggestible under the influence of LSD because conscientiousness is related to ego control, and LSD has been shown to have therapeutic benefits resulting from the disintegration of users egos while under the influence of the drug. LSD has the ability to enhance suggestibility in therapeutic environments with the majority of patients, especially those individuals who are trait conscientious. This is a result of LSD's ability to temporarily suspend the human desire to maintain control of the mind and the environment.

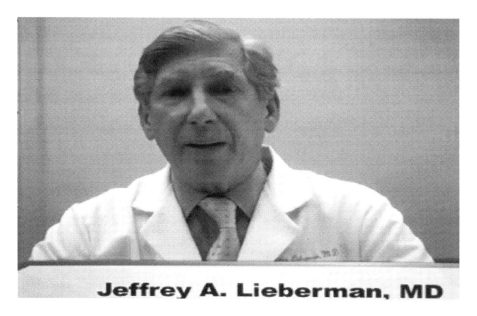

Jeffrey A. Lieberman, MD

(Our Amazing World, 2015)

Video of a psychiatrist discussing the use of psychedelic drugs used for psychotherapy. He elaborates on proposals for using psychedelic drugs in modern medicine and the necessity of standardizing the use of these drugs as treatments for psychological disorders.

Chapter 11: Ergot

Ergot is a plant disease caused by the fungus Claviceps purpurea on rye (University of Hawaii, 2016). Ergot forms on a single grain of rye, and it replaces the grain with a dark sclerotium, which forms after its sexual stage in the spring. The sexual stage consists of a mass of fungal tissue or stroma in which asci and ascospores are produced. The true nature of this fungus was not fully understood until the mid-nineteenth century when it was discovered to be a fungus and not part of the actual rye plant. Ergot is commonly found on rye, but the fungal disease also appears on other grains. The ergot stage of the development of the fungus contains a number of compounds that are important to the pharmaceutical industry. The number of compounds varies with plant species, and the mycotoxins that can be fatal when consumed. The symptoms of ergotism have been recorded for thousands of years, and the disease afflicted many individuals during the Middle Ages. Ergot is the original source in which the alkaloids necessary to produce LSD were first isolated by Albert Hoffman.

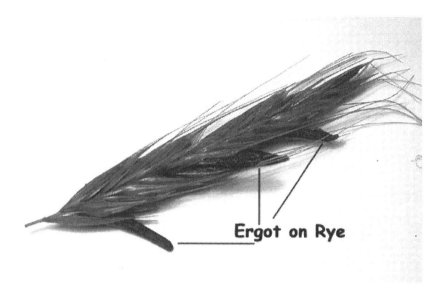

Ergot on Rye

(University of Hawaii, 2016, p. 1)

This image shows how ergot fungus grows on the individual grains of rye.

Ergotism is now rare because there is a screening of rye seeds in which a flotation system using 30% potassium chloride is poured on the rye seeds and stirred (University of Hawaii, 2016). This process results in the seeds infected with ergot rising and floating, and, then, they are skimmed off. To further decrease the amount of ergot formation in rye crops, fields are deeply plowed following a rye harvest, so ergot will not have the opportunity to germinate. Crop rotation can also be used to minimize the growth of ergot, and, to date, there has never been a strain of rye that has been developed that is completely resistant to the fungus.

In the 1930s, scientists at the Rockefeller Institute in New York determined the chemically active ingredients in ergot or ergot alkaloids, and they isolated and characterized the nucleus common with the alkaloids and name it lysergic acid. Albert Hoffman discovered LSD in the late 1930s when he was studying one of the derivatives of lysergic acid in which he produced a by-product of it and named it LSD (May, 1998). He stopped studying LSD for five years because he believed that there was no useful medical use for it. He repeated the synthesis of the drug in 1943 because he believed that he had missed something in his initial investigation, and he began self-tests of the substance and discovered its powerful psychedelic effects.

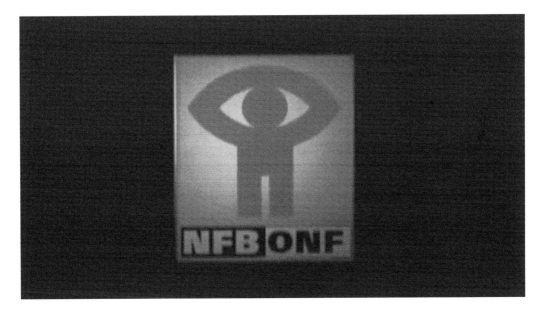

(Smith, 2012)

Video of Albert Hoffman discussing LSD and his view on the discovery of the drug. The video also discusses the history of the drug and the profound impact that it has had.

Chapter 12: Synthesizing LSD

Disclaimer: The synthesis of LSD is illegal, and it is a felonious activity that can lead to incarceration and cause psychosis in some users. LSD is popular, and people have been using the drug since it was first created and following it being classified as illegal in the mid-1960s. The synthesizing and manufacturing of it can be profitable and educational. Individuals that synthesize, sell, and use LSD are doing so illegally.

The synthesis of LSD should be done by a well-skilled chemist who has a background in organic chemistry, and individuals producing LSD should be well-trained prior to undertaking the task (Fester, 1996). LSD is much more difficult to synthesize than other conventional drugs like MDMA and methamphetamines, and, if done incorrectly, it can lead to death through poisoning the chemist or those who consume inferior synthesized products. Converting ergot, morning glory seeds, or Hawaiian baby woodrose seeds to LSD is complex but doable with some training and the correct instruction. LSD is one of the most powerful substances known to chemistry and synthesization of a single gram makes more than 10,000 doses, which can be easily absorbed through the skin. Therefore, the proper training, equipment, and precautions must be taken while synthesizing this drug.

Lysergic acid and the precursors to make LSD are extremely fragile, and they are susceptible to destruction from light, air, and heat (Fester, 1996). Good LSD synthesis cannot be done in a makeshift laboratory, and chemists looking to synthesize the drug properly should be attempting to do it with real laboratory equipment, which will require a minimum of a distilling kit with glass joints to synthesize reagents to a high-level of purity. Aspirators cannot be used, and chemists must be willing to spend $10,000 US or more for a proper vacuum pump and other essential equipment. The initial investment is high, but the return on good LSD produced can be enormous, especially if chemists avoid detection. Education for the synthesis of LSD is a must, and individuals planning to synthesize the drug should study at least a year of college-level organic chemistry in conjunction with some biology laboratory courses in which the use of chromatography is instructed to learn how to isolate biological substances. Chemists must familiarize themselves with sterile culture techniques, so they are able to cultivate ergot from rye fields. Chemists hoping to synthesize LSD in today's world must know how to isolate lysergic acid precursors from ergot, morning glory seeds, and Hawaiian baby woodrose, and they must be able to synthesize closely watched reagents like diethylamine in pure form.

The synthesis of LSD is a combination of farming, biology, biochemistry, and organic chemistry (Fester, 1996). To set up large-scale manufacture of LSD, chemists need a couple of acres of land to plant rye with Claviceps fungus, morning glories, or Hawaiian baby woodrose. Crops are then brought to laboratory sites for the biochemical phase of LSD manufacturing in which the isolation of lysergic alkaloids occurs, which are amides of lysergic acid. The lysergic acid molecule is what makes all known methods of LSD synthesis possible, and the commonality that all synthetic routes share to the synthesis of LSD is that they start with the naturally occurring alkaloids, the amide linkage is removed to produce lysergic acid, and, then, the lysergic acid is reacted with diethylamine to produce LSD.

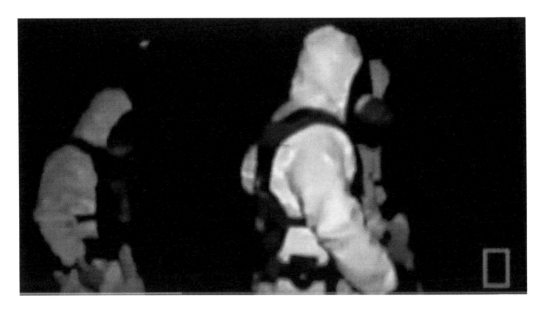

(HellaRatchet, 2013)

VIdeo showing the bust of an underground LSD lab. The man incarcerated and shown in the video discusses his logic behind producing LSD, and his opinion of the necessity of having LSD available, regardless of its illicitness, because of its pharmacologic properties and ability to help people psychotherapeutically.

Growing ergot fungus in a culture medium is nearly impossible for most strains of Claviceps fungus because it does not cooperate in this manner, so the logistical complications of growing rye infected with ergot are necessary to set up large-scale production of LSD (Fester, 1996). The majority of Claviceps fungi will not produce the necessary alkaloids required to make lysergic acid react with diethylamine to synthesize LSD. The most viable and safest sources of lysergic acid amides for the large-scale production of LSD will begin through growing ergot-infested rye, growing morning glories, or Hawaiian baby woodrose, which is required to obtain the raw material necessary to obtain lysergic compounds in an undetected manner. The best farming choice and the one that produces the purest LSD is the growth of ergot-infested rye because it does not contain other types of unwanted alkaloids from the clavine group that are present in both morning glory seeds and Hawaiian woodrose seeds, which can result in a contaminated finished product without the correct steps used to remove them. Ergot is not present in most rye crops because of modern day farming techniques, but there has not been a complete elimination of the fungus from rye crops to date. Therefore, ergot can still be collected from rye fields all over the world in small quantities, and it can generally be found around the edges of rye fields on contemporary farms and easily collected. Ergot collection is a necessary first step for individuals to grow their own ergot invested rye patches, and, after the collection of a few dozen heads of ergot, chemists will have enough Claviceps fungus to grow their own infested patches of rye.

For individuals to grow ergot successfully, they must understand the life cycle of the Claviceps fungus, which grows on the rye plant until it matures in the winter (Fester, 1996). Then, ergot falls of the rye plant and lies on the top of the soil until it matures and deposits spores into the air in spring when the weather becomes warmer. When spores land on the flower of the rye plant, they germinate and take over the flower by extracting nutrients from the plant. Chemists need to apply their biological science skills by germinating the spores in a sterile culture medium and spraying them onto their rye plants just as they are flowering to ensure a heavy infestation of ergot. This method has been used for nearly one hundred years with great success in the commercial production of ergot, and the yields of ergot are generally as high as one hundred pounds per acre, which could easily supply a chemist with enough of lysergic alkaloids for the synthesis of LSD for a decade or more.

Following the farming phase of LSD production, the harvest of ergot will be reduced to a size that is more convenient to handle in a laboratory setting (Fester, 1996). Two hundred pounds or ninety-one kilograms of ergot will yield about one pound or .45 kilograms of lysergic acid amides, which is worth several million dollars if moved wholesale when synthesized into LSD. This is one of the most challenging phases for chemists because properly extracting the lysergic acid amides requires a large amount of solvents. Chemists will need several 55-gallon drums of solvent, and the extraction must be done in a rural area for increased safety and to avoid detection resulting from the aroma. During the extraction phase, lysergic molecules are very unstable, so there is a window in which the lysergic amides can be synthesized into high-quality LSD because once they are released from ergot they can be easily damaged by light, heat, air, and poor handling. The first step of extraction involves grinding of the ergot, and, once this has begun, the lysergic molecules are unstable. Then, the ergot is moistened with a solvent for the defatting phase of extraction, which is an especially important phase in the isolation of pure alkaloids. If this phase is not done properly, the fats and oils present in the ergot will result in an emulsion forming during the extraction of the alkaloid, which leads to an inferior amide extract. The defatting phase can be easily done with common and easily available solvents like hexane, petroleum ether mineral spirits, or naphtha. Once the fats are removed from the ergot, the lysergic alkaloids can be extracted from the crop. The next phase involves removing the lysergic amides from the plant material to extract them into a solvent, which involves free basing the salt from the former phase in a solvent of chloroform or using magnesia as the basing agent with a solvent of ethyl ether or benzene. The second method is better and yields about 25% more lysergic amides being separated from the plant material at the end of the phase. During the extraction phase, the extract must be protected from light, and, for large scale operations, one can monitor the rate of extraction by using a black light because the lysergic amides fluoresce in a bluish color.

The next phase involves evaporating the extracted solvent using a vacuum in which the product must not be exposed to light or to heating above 105 degrees Fahrenheit or 40 degrees Celsius (Fester, 1996). When the chloroform in the original volume has been reduced to one-fifth of its original volume, the solvent must be diluted with ether. It is difficult to extract alkaloids from pure chloroform. The transfer of alkaloids into a tartaric-acid solution is much more efficient when the solution is predominantly ether, and benzene can also be substituted for ether at this stage. Ether is preferred at this stage, but it can draw attention from governments because any purchases of it that exceed twenty five gallons have to be reported to national governments.

The alkaloids are then extracted from the ether solution into a decimolar tartaric acid in water, which results in the alkaloids forming a salt with the tartaric acid and leaving the unwanted plant compounds in the ether (Fester, 1996). The extraction should be repeated four times with a volume of tartaric acid solution that is one-seventh the volume of the ether solution. Fresh tartaric acid must be used for each extraction, and, if emulsion forms, a bit of alcohol should be added to the solution. Tartaric acid is preferred for this phase because it is stable in light, but a .2N sulfuric acid solution can also be used as long as precautions are taken to protect the solution from exposure to light. Tartaric acid solution containing the alkaloids should be free-based with ammonia, and the ammonia should be added with vigorous stirring until the pH level reaches between 8 and 8.5. High pH levels must be avoided because it results in racemization, which causes an inactive iso form of lysergic acid. The free-based alkaloids should be extracted from the water solution into ether, and it should be repeated four times with a volume of ether one-fourth to that of water. Combined ether extracts from the solution should be dried over some magnesium sulfate that has been previously moistened with ether to prevent it from absorbing the alkaloids during the drying process. The ether should be evaporated under a vacuum until a residue of alkaloids remains, which must be immediately transferred to a freezer.

Once the amides have been extracted in a pure form from ergot, work should be undertaken to convert it to LSD (Fester, 1996). Possession of lysergic amides, if caught by the authorities, shows strong intent to synthesize LSD, and possession of lysergic acid and ergine are prohibited because they are considered to be controlled substances. There are several methods to produce LSD from lysergic amides, but the method chosen will most likely depend on the availability of chemicals to chemists. Methods using anhydrous hydrazine are preferable and is required if one is to use the procedure patented by Albert Hoffman, but the chemical is hard to obtain and heavily monitored by governments. It is possible to make anhydrous hydrazine from raw materials, but it requires a nitrogen atmosphere to avoid detonation. Hydrazine is also highly poisonous and toxic, and it can corrode and burn tissue. For Hoffman's method, three main precautions must be taken: water cannot be included at all in the reaction, the solvent cannot be exposed to light so work should be done under a dim red darkroom bulb, and the reaction must be done in a nitrogen atmosphere. All methods that are used to synthesize LSD from lysergic amides require the proper laboratory equipment, chemicals, and training. All stages LSD production must be preplanned from the collection of ergot to the synthesis phase, but, once the ergot extraction phase begins, the solution that is worked with is unstable and can be easily damaged. Also, the chemicals that are required to synthesize LSD can be unstable under certain conditions, so planning and training are a must to synthesize good, pure

LSD. There have been many books written on the synthesis of LSD, but "Practical LSD Manufacture" is recommended because the author offers detailed explanations regarding the different synthesis methods available to produce LSD and instruction on how to make some of the necessary chemicals, which are monitored by governments, from other readily available raw materials that are not overseen.

Once synthesized LSD is quite stable and can be stored for decades in the right conditions. Ideally, it would be best to synthesize lysergic amides as soon as possible following their extraction from ergot, but, if they are stored in a freezer, it is possible to synthesize smaller batches of LSD over a period of time. This would permit individuals who have access to university, private, and government laboratories to synthesize small batches of LSD in ideal conditions if they had the correct chemicals available to them before synthesis is attempted. The vast majority of the equipment needed for proper synthesis of LSD is available for sale from laboratory supply stores and online. This, however, can draw detection if one is not cautious. The advantage to synthesizing in an industrial laboratory setting is that the purity of the LSD synthesized could be potentially higher and the possibility in the process would decrease. It is possible to develop a good clandestine laboratory for large-scale LSD production with the right planning, knowledge, and money. This is clearly for profit, and the risks are large. There are many individuals, however, that use psychedelics in a ritualistic manner, and many of them are interested in synthesizing the drug for therapy and personal use.

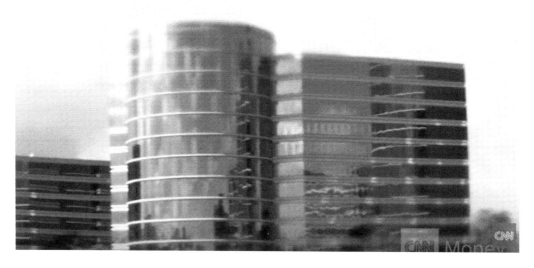

(CNNMoney, 2015)

Video discussing how LSD and other hallucinogens have assisted individuals in creating disruptive technology.

Reference Citations

Allen, P., Laroi, F., McGuire, P., and Aleman, A. (2008). The hallucinating brain: A review of the structural and functional neuroimaging studies of hallucinations, *Neuroscience and Behavioral Reviews*, 32(1), p. 175-191.

Archaesoup Productions (2016). Hidden Histories: Humans and Hallucinogens. Retrieved online from: https://www.youtube.com/watch?v=iJwyyBR9psI.

Brit Lab (2015). What Does LSD Do To Your Brain? Retrieved online from: https://www.youtube.com/watch?v=LJbrLSU2Tk4.

Brainwaves.com (2016). Your Brain and What it Does. Retrieved online from: http://www.brainwaves.com/.

Carhart-Harris, R., Kaelen, M., Bolstridge, M., Williams, T. Williams, L. , Underwood, R., Feilding, A., and Nutt, D. (2016). The paradoxical psychological effects of lysergic acid diethylamide, Psychological Medicine, 46(1), p. 1279-1290.

Carhart-Harris, R., Kaelen, M., Whalley, M., Bolstridge, M., Feilding, A., and Nutt, D. (2015). LSD enhances suggestibility in healthy volunteers, *Psychopharmacology*, 232(1), p. 785-794.

Carthart-Harris, R., Muthukumaraswamy, S., Roseman, L., Kaelen, M., Droog, W., Murphy, K., Tagliazucchi, E., Schenberg, E., Nest, T., Orban, C., Leech, R., Williams, L., Williams, T., Bolstridge, M., Sessa, B., McGonigle, J., Sereno, M., Nichols, D., Hellyer, P., Hobden, P., Evans, J., Singh, K., Wise, R., Curran, H., Feilding, A., and Nutt, D. (2016). Neural correlates of the LSD experience revealed by multimodal neuroimaging. Retrieved online from: http://www.pnas.org/content/113/17/4853.

CNNMoney (2015). Can LSD make you a billionaire? Retrieved online from: https://www.youtube.com/watch?v=jz9yZFtRJjk.

Devianart (2016). Tripping on LSD. Retrieved online from: http://derklox cloxboy.deviantart.com/journal/Tripping-on-LSD-part-1-of-2-231346037.

DNews (2014). How Do Magic Mushrooms Expand Your Mind? Retrieved online from: https://www.youtube.com/watch?v=BdVgQQIiZF0.

DNews (2015). Why do we hallucinate? Retrieved online from: https://www.youtube.com/watch?v=K1CUdLfGjBU.

Fester, U. (1996). Practical LSD Manufacture. Retrieved online from: https://files.shroomery.org/cms/5841102-practicallsd-UncleFester.pdf.

Galactic Scholar Consciousness (2013). Ayahuasca and the Brain. Retrieved online from: https://www.youtube.com/watch?v=aufjjU0EYxk.

Gasser, P., Holstein, D., Michel, Y., Doblin, R., Yazar-Klosinki, B., Passie, T., and Brenneisen, R. (2014). Safety and Efficacy of Lysergic Acid Diethylamide-Assisted Psychotherapy for Anxiety Associated With Life-threatening Diseases, *The Journal of Nervous and Mental Disease*, 202(1), p. 512-520.

Ghent University (2016). Serotonin. Retrieved online from: http://users.belgacom.net/neurobiology/serotonin.htm.

Hallucinogen. (2016). In *Encyclopedia Britannica*. Retrieved from http://academic.eb.com.contentproxy.phoenix.edu/levels/collegiate/article/38956.

HellaRatchet (2013). Real LSD Lab. Retrieved online from: https://www.youtube.com/watch?v=KokbQBpMh6o.

Herballove (2016). Youth Impotence: Caused by Ecstasy. Retrieved online from: http://www.herballove.com/guide/youth-impotence-caused-ecstasy.

Iaria, G., Fox, C., Scheel, M., Stowe, R., and Barton, J. (2010). A case of persistent visual hallucinations of faces following LSD abuse: A functional Magnetic Resonance Imaging Study, *Neurocase*, 16(2), p. 106-118.

Intergalactic (2010). Inside LSD. Retrieved online: https://www.youtube.com/watch?v=3sl4y-_CYsE.

Intergalactic (2010). Inside LSD Part 2. Retrieved online: https://www.youtube.com/watch?v=TqX7jcNcldw&list=PLEAD71609A00AE2B3.

Karst, M., Halpern, J., Bernateck, M., and Passie, T. (2010). The non-hallucinogen 2-bromo-lysergic acid diethylamide as preventative treatment for cluster headaches: An open, non-randomized case series, *Cephalalgia*, 30(10), p. 1140-1145.

LSD. (2016). In *Encyclopedia Britannica*. Retrieved from: http://academic.eb.com.contentproxy.phoenix.edu/levels/collegiate/article/49184.

Manford, M. & Andermann, F. (1998). Complex visual hallucinations: Clinical and neurobiological insights, *Brain*, 121(1), p. 1819-1841.

May, P. (1998). Lysergic Acid Diethylamide. Retrieved online from: http://www.chm.bris.ac.uk/motm/lsd/lsd.htm.

Multidisciplinary Association for Psychedelic Therapy (2014). Legalizing Psychedelic Therapy. Retrieved online from: https://www.youtube.com/watch?v=Oq80S9JOvT8.

National Institute of Drug Abuse (2016). Brain pathways are affected by drugs of abuse. Retrieved online from: http://gatest.iqscloud.net/publications/addiction-science/why-do-people-abuse-drugs/brain-pathways-are-affected-by-drugs-abuse.

Our Amazing World (2015). Top American Psychiatrist Jeffrey Lieberman Calls for Classic Hallucinogen Research. Retrieved online from: https://www.youtube.com/watch?v=4Qg6hABPxSY.

Quigley, A. and Waun, J. (2011). Lysergic Acid Diethylamide. The Gale Encyclopedia of Medicine. (Vol. 5, p. 2704-2705). Detroit: Cengage Learning.

Royal Society of Chemistry (2015). Lysergic acid diethylamide. Retrieved online from: http://www.chemspider.com/Chemical-Structure.5558.html.

Royal Society of Chemistry (2015). 2-Bromo-LSD. Retrieved online from: http://www.chemspider.com/Chemical-Structure.9765.html.

Santos, R., Osorio, F., Crippa, J., Riba, J., Zuardi, A., and Hallak, J. (2016). Antidepressive, anxiolytic, and antiaddictive effects of ayahuasca, psilocybin and lysergic acid diethylamide (LSD): a systematic review of clinical trials published in the last 25 years, *Therapeutic Advances in Psychopharmacology*, 6(3), p. 193-214.

Schindler, E., Dave, K., Smolock, E., Aloyo, V., and Harvey, J. (2012). Serotonergic and dopaminergic distinctions in the behavioral pharmacology of DOI and LSD, *Pharmacology, Biochemistry, and Behavior*, 101(1), p. 69-76.

Schmid, Y, Enzler, F., Gasser, P., Grouzmann, E., Preller, K., Vollenweider, F., Brenneisen, R., Muller, F., Borgwardt, S., and Liechti, M. (2015). Acute Effects of Lysergic Acid Diethylamide in Healthy Subjects, *Biological Psychiatry*, 78(1), p. 544-553.

Smith, K. (2012). Hofmann's Potion - Albert Hofmann LSD Documentary. Retrieved online from: https://www.youtube.com/watch?v=OpSLjdPiSH8.

TheLipTV (2016). LSD Brain Scan Reveals Stunning Info. Retrieved online from: https://www.youtube.com/watch?v=zJR19GOb5yQ.

Udacity (2015). Psilocybin side effects: Intro to Psychology. Retrieved online from: https://www.youtube.com/watch?v=xYUgNS_lbbk.

University of Hawaii (2016). Ergot of Rye. Retrieved online from: http://www.botany.hawaii.edu/faculty/wong/BOT135/LECT12.HTM.

Walacea (2015). Walacea: Crowdfunding video for Worlds first LSD Brain Imaging
    Study. Retrieved online from:
    https://www.youtube.com/watch?v=iiQNdYqboYM.

WebMD (2016). Cluster Headaches. Retrieved online from:
    http://www.webmd.com/migraines-headaches/guide/cluster-headaches.

Williams, S. (2015). LSD Addiction and Recovery Facts. Retrieved online from:
    http://www.recovery.org/topics/lsd-facts/.

70881160R10051